Table of Contents

1. Introduction
2. Staying Home
3. Assisted Living Facilities
4. Nursing Homes
5. Cleanliness
6. Appearances
7. Christian Facilities
8. Bathtubs?
9. Laundry
10. Clothing - What to Bring
11. Jewelry
12. Safety and Restraints
13. Incontinence
14. Resuscitate/DNR/Living Will/Etc.
15. Power of Attorney
16. Job Descriptions: Who Does What?
17. The Little Things?
18. Mind Tapes
19. Family
20. Alzheimer's
21. Nurse Consultants

22. Abuse

23. Angels

A note from the author

Mary Stormont holds a BS degree from Montana State University, as well as an Associate Degree in Nursing from Rock Valley College in Rockford, IL. She has worked over the years in numerous medical facilities in several states, and her experience covers all areas of nursing, but her primary interest lies in geriatric care.

She has acted as county Home Health Coordinator, charge nurse, and as Director of Nursing in various facilities, but Nursing Homes have always been her primary interest. This is a compilation of observations and ideas that have been gathered over the years as she worked in these various nursing settings.

The information presented here should be very useful for the resident as well as the family member facing the nursing home situation in their lives. The nursing home is not a "warehouse", or the "end" – it is simply another environment, another aspect of our lives. While not all of us will ultimately enter a nursing home, for those of us who will, there are numerous ways to make the experience more positive and rewarding.

Mary presents thoughts, ideas, and recommendations to enhance this environment and to make the nursing home experience all that it can be for yourself and/or your loved ones, and presents them here in a quick and easy to read style. You may cry, you may smile, but you will certainly gain some valuable knowledge from this book. Enjoy!

Myrna Mink, MSN, LE
Former Nursing Professor, Seattle Pacific University

Choosing A Nursing Home And Living With Your Choice

by Mary Stormont BS, RN

Copyright 1999 by Mary Stormont BS, RN

All Rights Reserved

This ebook is licensed for your personal enjoyment only. This ebook may not be re-sold or given away to other people. If you would like to share this ebook with another person, please purchase an additional copy for each recipient. If you're reading this ebook and did not purchase it, or it was not purchased for your use only, then please purchase your own copy. Thank you for respecting the hard work of this author.

All names have been changed to protect privacy except for that of my son, Sean, and my good friend, Myrna.

1. Introduction

I saw a bumper sticker one day that read "Be good to your children for they will pick your nursing home!" At first I laughed, as I supposed it was designed to make me do, but later I began to reflect on just what it had really said, and it wasn't so funny anymore. In a way, it is a true saying, but as the significance of the saying struck home, I began to reflect on the conception most people have of nursing homes in general, especially the elderly. And then it came to me that most people haven't the foggiest idea what nursing homes are all about, how they operate, or even how to go about choosing one, should the need arise.

Now, while I don't consider myself an expert, I do have what I feel are the necessary qualifications to at least present an intelligent and realistic view on the subject, having spent the majority of my nursing years in nursing homes - and loving them, I might add. Dealing with the elderly has been one of the most positive experiences in my life - they are wonderful! Ah! The stories they can tell - but that is another subject altogether.

I would simply like to present what I feel are the best ways to pick a nursing home - and then live with your decision, making life in that environment the most rewarding and positive that it can be. And trust me, life in a nursing home CAN be rewarding and enjoyable. But this experience, like most others in life that are positive, require a little work by the participants to ensure the outcome is as we would desire it to be. Let me show you how to chose, and then live with your choice of a nursing home.

2. Staying Home

If you are reading this, you probably are facing somewhat of a dilemma. Mom has been at home, either living with you, or living in her own home, but you don't feel you can keep her there any longer. You don't want to put her in a nursing home, but you just don't know what else to do. You have a life to lead, maybe you have children still at home, and a husband or wife who needs you also. So what can you do?

I want to put a few suggestions out here, just in case Mom really CAN still stay at home, wherever home may be.

First of all, family is always the best help there is, if they have time. In larger families, it is easier to do. You just take turns. I know of families that simply said "no way, Mom will stay at home if it kills us." (In some instances, it almost did, by the way.) Anyway, there were lots of older children in these families, and they took turns staying with Mom for one to two weeks at a time. It was hard, and their families had to adjust to their being away for a period of time, but since they all took turns at it, it wasn't a particularly difficult burden for any one individual. And they were able to keep their loved one at home until they died.

Check into home health agencies. Ask your doctor, or look in the phone book in the Yellow Pages. Home health agencies are everywhere, and you will be amazed at what services can be provided in the home, and Medicare and Medicaid often will pay the entire cost. So don't despair until you have checked this aspect out.

Sometimes you can hire help privately to stay with Mom full time, depending on how much help Mom needs. This can get expensive, but then you have to weigh the cost against Mom's desire to stay at home, and what you can afford. Factor everything in to arrive at what you can and can't do.

I have seen families simply refuse to put Mom in a nursing home. There were only one or two family members willing and able to take care of her at home, and they literally almost killed themselves doing it. Sometimes it is simply too much for one or two people to handle, and you have to face that if it applies to you. I know it is hard, especially when your loved one says "I won't go to a nursing home. I want to stay in my own home. I can take care of myself. (You KNOW she/he can't!) You just don't want me around anymore. You are being selfish, and after all I did for you ..." The elderly can be very manipulative if they want to be at times. And they are sincere! They DON'T want to leave their homes. None of us do. But sometimes we don't have a choice. You know that old saying, "Life is what happens to you when you have other plans"? Well, it happens to young people too. What about the quadriplegic who accidentally fell off the roof while patching some shingles, and now is in a nursing home? Or the motor vehicle accident victim who is now on a respirator for the rest of his life? Or the Down's Syndrome child who has reached his twenties, but is no longer able to live at home? Sometimes, it just happens. We didn't plan it, we don't like it, we don't want it, but there is nothing we can do about it.

So don't keep Mom at home at the expense of your health and mental well being. And for heaven's sake, DON'T feel guilty about your decision. You do what you have to do, and what is best for ALL concerned, and sometimes the health and well being of the family must come before the desires of one individual.

Just remember, as I will say repeatedly — nursing homes aren't warehouses, or torture chambers, they are simply alternate environments. They are not by definition BAD, only DIFFERENT. I have talked to residents who wished they had gone to the nursing home years earlier, but they hated the thought, and expected the worst. They just didn't know.

One more thing. The elderly who remain at home, alone or with one or two family members, often are truly deprived of essential socialization in that environment. It is not done intentionally, it just happens. In the nursing home, they are exposed once again to other individuals with potentially similar interests and ideas. There is opportunity there to visit with others, and this keeps their minds younger and more alert.

So don't be afraid of the nursing home, and don't carry that big load around on your shoulders because you have made the decision to put Mom there, possibly against her wishes. You have a life, and you have to live too. And you can't be much support to Mom if you are dragged down emotionally and spiritually because of the situation. You just do the best you can with what you have.

3. Assisted Living Facilities

First, let me explain that the standard term "Nursing Home" doesn't really apply any more. There are several types of facilities out there to choose from, and perhaps a brief explanation of each is appropriate here.

"Assisted Living" facilities are fairly common, but often hard to find. These facilities are for those residents who are able to perform most ADL's (activities of daily living) by themselves, but perhaps need assistance with their bathing, taking their medications, choosing their clothing for the day, etc. Residents of these facilities must be ambulatory, and able to exit the facility on their own in case of emergencies. In reality, living here is very similar to living in an apartment, but a registered nurse is on staff for emergencies, and there is daily supervision and assistance as needed. On the plus side, these facilities are usually more home like in atmosphere, smaller, and in general the most pleasant on first inspection. If the potential resident simply can't live alone at home anymore, these are a great way to go. Very often, pets are allowed such as dogs, cats, or song birds. These facilities often offer exercise classes, chapel, and numerous other activities, but not always. If these activities are important to you, be sure to check if they are offered in the one you are considering.

Medications in these facilities are not always given by nursing staff. Aides (or personal care attendants, as they are often called) can be trained to administer medications when they have been previously set up by a nurse. Personally, I feel that this is one of the biggest drawbacks to these types of facilities. Aides are simply not trained in the use and side effects of medications, only on how and when to administer them. This leaves the door wide open for medication errors. Again, this is only my opinion, but I have worked in these facilities, and I have seen what can happen. If Mom is on a lot of different medications, you might want to check as to who will be giving the x meds - a nurse or an aide. If medications given are very few, and often no more than a daily multivitamin, maybe this isn't a big concern for you. But if it is, you might want to skip the assisted living facility, and continue your search on to the standard nursing home.

Another consideration - because there often is not a nurse in attendance at all times, emergencies such as sudden illnesses or accidents can be expensive, because they will most likely involve a trip to the emergency room, often by ambulance.

However, if Mom simply can't be trusted in the kitchen any more, (perhaps she forgets to turn off the stove?) or she can't remember to eat, or simply can't remember just what to do next, these are a great environment. One thing to remember though - often, if Mom's condition should deteriorate drastically, she may not be able to stay in that type of facility. Be sure to check out the facility's policies thoroughly if this will be important to you down the line. Remember that Assisted Living Facilities are just that - assisted living. They do not furnish standard nursing care as do the standard nursing homes. For special needs, however, most states have home health programs that allow for "home" visits (their home being the facility). When considering one of these facilities, be sure to ask if this service is available. The cost is often covered by Medicare when the visits are physician ordered, and most doctors are more than willing to participate in the program because it ensures better patient care.

I said these facilities are sometimes difficult to locate, because they are often not listed in the Yellow Pages, and are usually privately operated. Check with your doctor, the local home health agencies, and ask around - usually someone knows someone who knows someone who is living in a facility such as this, and can give you a place to start your search. If all else fails, call your State Department of Health. All facilities such as these must be licensed, and the department will have a listing of all of them in the state.

4. Nursing Homes

Ah - the standard "Nursing Home"! Strikes terror into many hearts - but needlessly, let me reassure you. They really are not torture chambers, or warehouses, or anything remotely like them. They are simply a different environment than what most of us are used to.

To begin, let me say that I have worked in numerous nursing homes, both as an aide and as a registered nurse. My opinion was the same regardless of the job I was performing.

I worked in several different types of nursing homes: one, in Pennsylvania, was for residents who stated upon admission that should their condition deteriorate to the point of death, they did not wish any extraordinary measures taken to prolong their lives, and signed a statement upon admission to that effect. Others offer standard nursing care only, with nothing extra (excluding activities, which I believe all nursing homes have as required by state laws.) And still others have a "rehabilitation center" as either an integral part of their facility, or as a major sideline, so to speak. They each have their place, and all three are necessary in our society. Depending on your needs, there will be one that is more suitable than another for you.

"Rehab Centers" or " Convalescent Centers" are kind of the new thing these days. Theses facilities offer intensive therapies, often on a daily basis, for different needs. They are often combined with the nursing home, to offer a range and variety of services. Whereas ten years ago post surgical patients often had a prolonged hospital stay, today these patients are often sent to recover at a nursing home, which incorporates numerous modalities for full recovery. There is a reason for this: MONEY. That's right, MONEY. Medicare and insurance companies reimburse, "big time" for therapies. This includes physical therapy, occupational therapy, and just about any other kind of therapy you can dream up. Did you know that physical therapists earn more money than registered nurses? The more therapy a facility can offer a resident, the more money the facility makes. So, this is good, and it is bad. Be aware of the differences, which I will try to explain.

On the plus side of this, for the post surgical patient who expects to return home, therapy is great. I am all for it. For instance, those recovering from a broken hip should have no fear of going to the nursing home to recover and learn, through therapy, how to ambulate again and regain their lives as they knew them. Knee replacements, back surgery, mild strokes, open heart surgery - all of these and numerous others are quite appropriate nursing home/rehab center placements. Patients there will benefit greatly from the therapies offered, recovery time is shortened dramatically, and they are often able to return home much sooner than they ever expected.

But consider carefully if you want Mom to have all this therapy if she is simply old and tired. Over ambitious therapists can do more harm than good. Doctors will often order therapy because someone suggests it, without really thinking it through. Remember that therapists bill by the visit - if they don't see Mom, they can't bill for it. Again, these visits are paid by Medicare and insurance companies, but the facilities are trying to maximize profits, and they will do it any way that they can. If, in your opinion, Mom would be better off just left alone to enjoy her time as she sees fit, don't go along with the therapy pitch. While it is true that many elderly people can benefit from some daily therapy, many others will never benefit from it, and it only ends up to be a mild form of torture for them. If you choose to go along with the therapy request, you might stipulate that if Mom is having a "bad day", or just not feeling well, she is NOT to have the therapy. Only family can really do anything about this situation. And nurses. Another subject for later on.

You may live in a small town, and "choosing" a nursing home for Mom might not be an option. There may be only one facility in the immediate area. Don't despair - I have found that over all, the smaller the community and the smaller the nursing home, the higher the overall quality of care in that home. These smaller homes offer a more home like environment overall, and most of the residents know each other and have for years. It is great.

OK - we now know that there are several different types of facilities to choose from. (And you thought this was going to be easy!) How do you actually pick a facility? Now comes the fun part!

5. Cleanliness

Clean. You want your loved one in a clean environment, right? Don't we all! This sounds like a fairly simple task - choosing a clean facility. I suppose it is fairly simple, in the end, but let me point out a few things to look for.
One of the first things you notice when you enter a facility, is odor. Does it reek of urine? Some facilities I have worked in seem to have a constant odor. Remember that housekeeping is separate from nursing, and sometimes it is simply a function of who the housekeeping staff is comprised of that week. If you visit a facility, and you notice a definite odor but you like everything else about the building, it might be an idea to visit the facility again in a week or two. Just because there is an odor one day, doesn't mean it will be present another day. Maybe the facility was really short staffed the day you came - maybe two or three house keepers failed to show up for work. You never know. If in doubt, ask the administrator about it. See what he/she says about the situation.
Never base your decision on the front lobby. Often these are beautiful, spacious rooms, decorated to the nines, and totally deceptive. They are modern, comfortable, clean-and not lived in. The real environment is beyond the doors, down the halls. Look in the corners. Are the corners clean? Check the bathrooms. Personally, I always thought if the bathrooms were clean, the place was in pretty good order in that respect. But you need to check not only visitor or staff bathrooms - sneak a look into a resident's bathroom. Ask a resident if you can take a look - most won't mind the intrusion at all, especially if you tell them why you are looking the place over.

Notice the glasses of residents who are wearing them. Are the lenses clean? Or is it a miracle if they can see anything at all? Glasses are often one of the most overlooked items in a nursing home. If the resident doesn't complain, it's just one of those things that, you know, if you aren't the one trying to see through them, you just don't notice. But it is another little way to gauge how much attention is being paid to the smaller, but still important aspects of everyday life.

Look at the faces of the residents. Are they clean? Or can you tell what each one had for lunch that day just by looking at their face? Are they wearing lunch on their clothing? Some people feel that wearing bibs at meals is degrading. Personally, I would prefer to wear a bib at a meal than wear my meal for the rest of the day on my blouse. (Which, incidentally, I have done). Some of us are a little sloppier than others, and it is not necessarily a function of old age! Bibs are optional. I am simply suggesting that you can also get an idea of cleanliness by looking at what residents are wearing - on their clothes as well as on their faces.

While you are observing the building (and checking the corners!), kind of casually glance at the fingernails of the residents, especially those residents who are more confused or lethargic. You know, those people who no longer visit with family, staff, or visitors. Are their fingernails neatly trimmed and clean, or is lunch under their nails as well as in their stomachs?

For those residents who smile at you as you pass by, are their teeth clean? Or do they look like you want to dive in with a new toothbrush and scrub?

Wheelchairs. Check out the wheelchairs! If the wheelchairs are clean, you can bet the rest of the facility isn't too far behind. Look closely at the arms and seats of the chairs in use. If they look a little crusty, mention it to a nurse or housekeeper. Wheelchairs are on a regular schedule to be cleaned, usually at night, and often by the night aides. While this is separate from housekeeping, it is a gauge of how closely attention is being paid to the little things around there.

Walk down the halls and take a look in the rooms. Are the beds neatly made? Are the wastebaskets empty, or at least not overflowing? (And speaking of wastebaskets, do they contain paper products or "toxic waste" that should never be left in a room? If it is something you don't recognize, it probably doesn't belong there.) Are the floors free of clutter? Do the rooms look inviting and comfortable? I personally would rather see a slightly cluttered room, full of treasures from home, than one that is so stark that it might as well be a hospital room. There is clean, and there is clutter. Remember that people LIVE in those rooms, and they should reflect that condition. Not necessarily immaculate, but an overall sense of cleanliness, at least.

Are the halls clear? They should be kept free of hampers, etc. unless the aides are doing rounds.

Are disposable gloves being used by housekeepers and nursing staff, including aides? Disposable gloves should be readily available, and they should be used during patient care, bathroom cleaning, etc.

Also remember that there are certain times of the day that are much busier than others. Early in the morning, residents are getting up, and general mayhem is in progress until after breakfast. If you expect to make a relaxed visit, don't do it in the morning. Come after lunch. Of course, if you really want to know the inner workings of the facility, the reverse is true - show up around 7:30 or 8:00 in the morning. You will learn what it is REALLY like! Just don't expect miracles at that hour. It takes time and effort to keep a facility clean and presentable. It doesn't just happen. If you are in doubt, make several visits over a period of days, and at different times. But remember that the nursing home is a residence for many people. You are there, inspecting their home. Remember that when you are visiting, and treat the residents with respect for their privacy, just as you would want to be treated if guests came to your house, uninvited. I do, however, think that surprise visits are probably the best for seeing what a facility is really like. If at all possible, check with someone who lives in the facility, or the family of someone that lives there. Have them go with you, or make plans to visit the resident, with the objective of "casing the joint". But don't try to fool anybody; if you are asked what you are doing there, be honest and tell them you are considering placing Mom in the facility, and you wanted to see what the building and routine were like.

I think it is a good idea to make several visits to each prospective building. Make one or two unannounced, and make an appointment to be given a guided tour. If you don't think you can remember everything you are looking for/at, make a checklist and take it with you. Don't be embarrassed by this - at least they will know you are serious in your endeavor.

You can always ask how the facility scored on their last visit from the state. They may or may not tell you, but if they are reputable, they will be honest and up front about this. The state visits facilities at least yearly, and gives them written notice of any deficiencies found. These must be corrected before the next visit. It is true that often the state will "nit-pick" over stupid (to my way of thinking) little things, but over all, if the facility is not up to par, it will not pass inspection. It is perfectly within your right to ask if it did. Another little thing - not necessarily to do with cleanliness, but along the same lines - how are the staff dressed? Are the nurses wearing clean uniforms or scrubs? Some facilities allow their staff to wear street clothes, in an effort to make the environment more "home like". This is fine - but are they clean and neat? Are sweat pants the order of the day? (I don't think so!! Inappropriate!) Are the aides dressed neatly? Gaudy makeup and jewelry is not appropriate for this environment, but again, if in doubt, ask the administrator. Some facilities have "dress down" days - maybe you happened to visit on one of these days.

And finally, don't be afraid to ask the residents how they feel about the facility. Do they think it is clean? Do they approve of how the staff is dressed? Ask them if they would recommend the facility to someone else? And be sure to ask several different residents. You can never go by just one opinion, and that applies to nearly any situation, not just nursing homes. If you don't know who to ask, stop an aide or a nurse and ask them who would be appropriate for you to visit with.

Remember that in the end, while you want the facility of your choice to be clean (immaculate might be a better descriptive word for most of us "picky" people!) the most important aspect of the environment is the care of the residents. We want our selection to be the perfect one, the best there is available, where our loved one is going to stay. But I don't care if the building literally shines and you can see your reflection on the bathroom sink, if resident's have dirty fingernails and faces, and the wheelchairs are a little crusty, I wouldn't want to put Mom in that facility. I would far rather have the bathroom not quite so clean and have the residents sparkling. Patient care is the true "name of the game", and it had better come first.

6. Appearances

I want to point out one little thing here. Don't let the general appearance of the building sway you in your final decision. There are some really beautiful new buildings out there, and your first thought will probably be "Yup! This is what I want for Mom. All the newest and the best." But remember, you are really looking for superior nursing and personal care, not appearances.

One of the best facilities I ever worked in was so old, I was actually dismayed when I walked in the door to apply for a position as charge nurse. The rooms were small, and dark. There were no private bathrooms; there were community bathrooms on each hall. There was no whirlpool. There were no nice lawns - in fact, there was hardly any lawn at all. Only about three of the rooms had a view, and that was of the street. The rest looked out onto an alley, or had no outside window at all. There was no elevator, and it was a two story building, so a chair lift was in use for those who could not manage stairs on their own. There was no air conditioning. And I admit, it was far from the cleanest facility I was ever in. But the staff was so friendly! After being in that atmosphere for about fifteen minutes, I realized that it is the people that make a facility, not the outward appearance. The nursing care was excellent, and because of the friendly atmosphere, residents were relaxed and comfortable. The cooks were so helpful, they made special meals and snacks for those who requested them, any time they wanted. It was like an open cafeteria for those residents that they never had to pay extra for. Also, remember that just because a facility appears somewhat dark, and maybe to us, gloomy, the elderly often prefer darker environments. It is more restful for them, and sometimes the brighter lights seem to hurt their eyes after a period of time. You are not looking for a hospital, you are looking for a home.

On the other hand, I have worked in relatively new facilities that were really state of the art. They were beautiful, inside and out. Everything was spacious and well lighted, and even the corners were shining, the place was so clean. There was definitely no odor, anywhere. The nursing care was excellent. It was spotless. It was professional. It was like an institution in that place. And I didn't like working there. It was SO professional, it had lost it's home-like atmosphere. True, the residents were all well cared for, but the facility lacked all the elements that make a building more of a HOME. Given a choice, if I had to pick one of these two facilities to put my mother in, I would probably have to go with the older one, knowing what I do about the inside workings of the various facilities.

Now, if Mom has become one of those elderly people that either refuses, or simply no longer is able to communicate, and seems to always be off in her own world, then probably the newer facility would be my choice. Or if she has Alzheimer's. You have to look at the overall picture, and weigh the pros and cons of each situation. And remember that just because a facility is new, I am NOT saying it isn't as good as an older one. I AM saying that just because a facility is old, doesn't mean it may not provide excellent care. (One other thing, if cost is a factor in nursing home placement, often the older facilities are substantially cheaper.)

Again, in the end, the best way to tell what daily life in a facility is like, is to simply talk to the residents who live there. They have no reason to lie to you, so when you visit, ask the nurses or the activities person to introduce you to several different residents for you to visit with. Or ask if you can just sit down with a cup of coffee in the dining room or maybe in one of the lounges where residents are congregated, and observe. Given enough time, you will either begin to relax or feel like you can't get out of there quick enough. (Although some individuals have such a horror of nursing homes, they can't get out quick enough no matter WHAT the facility if like!) Again, keep in mind that a nursing home is not a bad environment, it is simply a DIFFERENT environment.

7. Christian Facilities

I wanted to mention that there are facilities, usually nursing homes (as opposed to personal care centers) that are owned and operated by churches or Christian non-denominational organizations. These seem to be located mostly in the larger cities, but the ones I have seen were really a cut above the others, at least in appearance. I never was privileged to work in one (except as an aide while in nurse's training, and then I was working for an agency so only worked a couple of evening shifts). They operate on Christian principles, and I really enjoyed being in these facilities. For many people, knowing that it is a Christian nursing home is a very important factor, especially if church has always played a large part in their lives.

One of the most "posh" homes I visited had graduated levels of care, more so than the standard nursing homes. There were lovely brick duplexes across the spacious lawn from the main building. These were for sale, for a price that was fair and reasonable compared to other comparable duplexes in the city. But inside the living quarters, (which were VERY nice) call lights were installed everywhere. A person or couple could purchase the duplex, and were then assured their personal care for the rest of their lives. If they became unable to cook for themselves, but were still able to live at home alone, meals were brought from the main building. As they aged and their condition deteriorated to the point where it was no longer feasible to be living independently, they moved to a separate wing in the main building.

The next level was a wing of spacious apartments with private patios and small kitchenettes. There were large patio windows with full length drapes, and every apartment had a lovely private view of the grounds. And again, call lights throughout in case help was needed. If and when the resident required more supervision and care, they moved on to the next wing, which was the standard nursing home room.

But the beauty of the whole thing was there was only the initial purchase of the duplex itself. I think at that time, the price was around $50,000, if I remember correctly, and as long as the mortgage payments were made faithfully, there was never an additional charge to live anywhere in the facility. It was like buying a house or a condominium, but being assured that you would never have to move far again, or come up with more money down the road.

There are probably other facilities such as this one that are run by non-Christian organizations, though I have never seen one. But I wanted to be sure to point out that Christian run facilities are out there, for those who prefer them. They may be specified in the Yellow Pages, or you might ask your pastor about it. Sometimes they don't tell you in the Yellow Pages or advertisements that they are Christian owned and operated, so you will have to check it out if this is important to you.

8. Bathtubs?

I know, I know, bathtubs? Am I serious? Sure am. Every facility you look at should have at least one bathtub per hallway. If every room has a private bathroom, there will probably be a shower stall, a sink, and a toilet in each, with a separate shower/tub area located elsewhere, and it really doesn't matter where. However, there is a definite difference in tubs!

Usually, when you think of a bathtub, you think of the old standard tub we are all familiar with. In nursing homes, it usually sort of sticks out from a wall so it is accessible from both sides and the back. But the really neat tubs are a kind of therapy tub. They are usually made out of fiberglass, and are similar to a one person hot tub/whirlpool that are so popular today. There is a swivel chair with a hydraulic lift mechanism at the end of the tub, and the resident is transferred from the wheelchair (or just walks to this chair), is belted in for safety, then lifted up and over into the tub using the hydraulic lift. The resident does not lie down in the tub, but rather sits on a nice fiberglass seat, never getting out of the hydraulic lift chair itself. There are several jets surrounding the client, and a luxurious whirlpool bath is a piece of cake for even the most debilitated resident. In one nursing home where I worked, we had non-resi- dents coming in for prescribed whirlpools, usually related to back injuries or chronic leg problems. They loved that tub! We would fill the tub, put them in, turn on the jets, give them a call light, and come back in two hours unless called for earlier. That nursing home was pretty popular with some of the folks in town, not counting the residents! (I know that after hours, some of the staff even availed themselves of the luxury.)

Anyway, a whirlpool tub is not a necessity, by any means, but if Mom really prefers a tub bath to a shower, you might ask if they have a whirlpool tub available. If they say that they do, also be sure to clarify whether or not it is one of the old standard therapy whirlpools or one of these that I am describing. The standard therapy whirlpool baths are a tub designed primarily for soaking legs and feet only. You can't fit a whole body in the tub.

Another thing you will have to follow up on if Mom prefers the tub baths, is whether or not she is actually getting them. Again, we come back to the time factor, which is always in such short supply in facilities. Whirlpool baths take longer than showers, no matter how you do it, and the aides don't want to take the time for them. However, if Mom has a skin condition, a special foot problem, or some other medical reason that would really benefit from a whirlpool or soaking, have the doctor prescribe them, and they will get done. If she doesn't have any medical reason for them, you can still just tell the staff that she is to have one once a week, or maybe once every other week, with showers in between. You may have to follow up to be sure they are actually GIVING the whirlpool baths, but if they are, believe me, Mom will love them.

While you certainly don't want to base your facility selection on a whirlpool tub, it is one of those little things you might want to check on while you are looking. Hey, it might be the straw that tips the scales, if you get down to two facilities and you just can't make up your mind.

9. Laundry

Laundry is another one of those topics that simply never occur to many families, but is one of the more important aspects of the nursing home. All facilities offer laundry services as part of the standard care program. However, be aware that this is the best way for items of clothing to get lost. You know, the "Great Black Hole" you thought only existed where your kid's clothes and shoes were concerned? Not true! That "Hole" is alive and well in all nursing homes and personal care centers. First of all, if you elect to have the facility do Mom's laundry, be sure to mark EVERYTHING with indelible ink. Permanent markers. Sew labels in. Whatever it takes. And even then, be prepared to occasionally walk in and see one of Mom's flowered blouses on Greta who lives down the hall. This is simply a function of life in a nursing home. Aides or laundry personnel get in a hurry, and misplace items of clothing. I don't think it is ever done on purpose, but it does happen. And personally, I don't know of any way to prevent this from occurring occasionally. But if you notice it being a common happening, by all means, let the staff know you are upset, and you don't want to see it happen again! Remember, "the squeaking hinge gets the oil". So, squeak a little. When families complain, staff listens. After all, it is you paying their salary, one way or another. They are working for you, not the other way around.

Be aware that nursing home detergents are not as gentle as what you use for your personal laundry at home. They aren't very generous with the fabric softener either. Some facilities are better than others about this, but still, facility laundries are hard on clothing. They have to be - you never know for sure what is going into that load of clothes, and they don't do laundry by individual rooms or people. All the clothing gets thrown in together, and usually washed according to color. The larger the facility, the less sorting is done. Fabric doesn't last as long, thread rots away, buttons get lost and not replaced, etc. So what can you do to minimize the problem? If the clothing has few or no buttons, they can't come off and get lost, right? Zippers seem to last forever. Nylon is almost indestructible, and cotton has a pretty long life also. Avoid any wool items, for sure. And anything that needs to be dry cleaned - chances are they will end up in the common laundry, and who knows what they will be like when they come back! See the section on Clothing for further discussion on what types of clothing to provide.

The other option, which many families chose, is to do Mom's laundry yourself. This is a great idea if you live close enough, and have the time. By doing the laundry yourself, you can use any type of detergent you desire - and it probably won't be as harsh as what the facility uses. You can use all the fabric softener you wish. If buttons come off in the wash, you know where they came from, and can sew them back on. Fabrics that need special care can be laundered properly.

A few things to remember though, if you chose to do the laundry yourself; still, BE SURE TO MARK EVERY ITEM OF CLOTHING WITH PERMANENT MARKER. They can still be misplaced (somehow!) Second, have a laundry bag in the room (marked, of course!), make up a sign and tape it to the wall stating "family will do laundry". And be sure to tell the staff. Tell the charge nurse. Tell every aide that comes into the room. Make sure it is common knowledge that you will be doing the laundry. It may take awhile for everyone to get the message, but for the most part, the laundry will make it to the bag you have provided. By doing it yourself, it also seems to make a huge difference regarding whose drawers Mom's clothing ends up in. You do it yourself, you put it away yourself, and it always seems to end up in the right drawers and closet that way. Amazing!

Laundry really isn't that big of a deal, in the long run, but it can be just another one of those little "thorns" in daily life. And since there seem to be more than enough of the little devils, if even one can be eliminated, why not do it? So, my advice is, if you have the time, and it isn't too great a hardship for you, do the laundry yourself. You will be much happier, (and probably, so will Mom) in the end.

One more thing. If you decide to do the laundry, try convincing the administrator to lower your monthly bill accordingly. You may not get anywhere with this, but it is worth a try. After all, you will be paying for a service you are not using - you should get a proportionate deduction in the monthly bill, right? It probably isn't worth arguing over but any way to save a nickel - or in this case, several nickels!

10. Clothing - What to Bring

Just a little bit here about what types of clothing you should bring for Mom to the nursing home or personal care center. While I am sure there will be certain favorite outfits that simply have to go to the facility with her, consider the new environment when thinking about clothing. A lot will depend on what kind of physical condition the new resident is in: is she bed/wheelchair bound? Can she dress herself, or does she need help in the morning? Can she take herself to the bathroom, or does she need assistance? Can she walk by herself? These are all factors to be considered when talking about clothing.

For the most part, I think sweats are the best thing ever to come down the pike, so to speak, when talking about nursing home clothing. They are soft, they are warm (and most elderly people are constantly cold!), they are easy to put on and take off, they have no buttons to lose or zippers to get caught, they come in attractive styles and colors, and they prevent the wearer from ever being "exposed" inadvertently. You can dress them up or down, and are always appropriate. I have known some residents whose entire wardrobes consisted of sweat suits.

For special occasions, you might have one or two good outfits in the closet, or keep them at home and bring them in as needed. Some elderly really reject sweats; they want dresses or dress pants (for men), white shirts and ties. In the end, if the wearer isn't comfortable with what she/he is wearing, their life will be miserable, so you can't force them to wear sweats just because you think they are better. But if you have the choice and the opportunity, go with sweats.

If Mom simply must wear dresses, consider shifts or caftans. Preferably with long sleeves, if you can find them. A lot of ladies prefer the "dusters", and these are fine, but unless they zip up the front, snaps and buttons can easily come undone, exposing the resident. The remedy for that, if you can get away with it, is to put them on backwards. They are just as comfortable, and exposure is greatly reduced.

If she won't wear sweats, by sure to bring a selection of sweaters. The elderly have a "lower thermostat" in general, than the rest of us, and they can become easily chilled in what to us is a pretty comfortable environment. Check her hands - if they are cool to the touch, she probably needs more covering for warmth. You often see people in nursing homes in wheelchairs, with lap robes over their knees. In some cases, it is for modesty, for instance if they are wearing a duster or a dress and their legs are exposed. In many cases, though, it is simply for warmth. Anything to conserve heat.

If you do bring a selection of sweaters, again, you might have to remind the staff to put them on Mom. Remember that the aides and nurses are usually moving at a pretty rapid pace, trying to get their work done, and they are probably sweating. It doesn't occur to them sometimes that Mom is sitting still, and she is cold. If it takes more than one reminder, so be it. Remember the "squeaking hinge" principle. It works!

Shoes. Depending on Mom's condition, shoes vary also. If Mom is bed/chair ridden, and no longer walks (except maybe to the bathroom) consider the terry slippers, or slipper socks. They have a latex or rubber sole or coating on the bottom, for better traction, but they are easily washed. Shoes get dirty, just like everything else. If they can be washed, it is a GREAT convenience. They are also very comfortable, and are seldom too tight, as laces can be over a period of time. If Mom still gets around pretty well, let her keep whatever shoes she is comfortable in. Canvas sneakers, or tennis shoes, are also good. Again, they have the non-slip sole for traction, but can be thrown in the washer if necessary. Traction is important in the nursing home, because most facilities do not have carpeting, for sanitary reasons. The floors are washed and waxed regularly, and this can lead to falls. Because the elderly are often cold, another good idea is undershirts, both for men and women. They may not seem like much, but they can make a real difference. Make sure you bring plenty of them - undershirts and underpants are two things you don't want to run out of! And speaking of underpants, I again recommend cotton, if at all possible. Cotton "breathes" better than nylon, and if the resident will be sitting a great deal of the time, it is healthier for them to be wearing cotton underwear.

Stockings are another important item. It may depend on what type of shoes you have talked Mom into, but if she will wear the terry slippers, try to talk her into thicker, cushioned, socks. Again, they are warmer. Many older residents will not give up their nylon stockings, even if they are only knee highs. And gentlemen often prefer those thinner, dress socks. They are better than nothing, but good cotton socks are best, if they will wear them.

A relatively new addition to the world of socks are "Smartwool" socks. They come in different weights and heights and are simply wonderful. They also come in lots of fun colors and patterns for both men and women. These wool socks don't itch, are machine washable, and are probably the warmest socks on the market. You might want to check them out on the internet. Do a search for "smartwool" and see what comes up.

Just be sure to try the shoes and socks on together before leaving Mom to daily life there. If they are new, be sure the shoes are not too tight with the socks on. I have seen residents that had to leave their shoes untied because their socks were too thick for the shoes. Also, if you can get the over-the-calf socks, or knee highs, they will be warmer than anklets.

Night wear can be whatever is comfortable and easy to get in and out of. Nightgowns are generally better than pajamas, if Mom will wear one. (For men, nightshirts are preferable to pajamas, but most men refuse to wear them.) Flannel is good, (again, it is warmer and usually pretty soft), but really, as long as they are warm at night, just about any kind will do. Remember that time is one of the most important factors for staff in nursing homes. They never seem to have enough of it. So the easier the clothing is to put on and take off, the better it is for everyone involved.

One more thing - don't forget to leave a winter coat in the closet for Mom, especially if you live in a cooler climate. You never know when something will come up, and she will have to go outside, for example an unanticipated visit to the doctor. She will feel better about being out in public if she has a regular coat. Otherwise, she will be bundled up in a blanket, which works fine, but just doesn't look as good. Also, along with the coat, how about a scarf or hat of some kind, and maybe a pair of gloves? Leave these items in the coat pockets, or they will probably be missed when the time comes that they are needed.

11. Jewelry

Most residents, when entering the nursing home, keep their wedding rings. And any costume jewelry is fine. I know of one lady who brought a huge jewelry case with her, and believe me, it was full! But it was all inexpensive jewelry, which is quite appropriate. Never bring valuables to a nursing home. Never. While it is sad, it is a fact that not everyone is honest. I have faith that the majority of staff in nursing homes are painfully honest, but it only takes one thief to cause a lot of grief, and you never know who they are, or where they are. Diamonds, expensive watches, etc. should always be left at home. You can bring them in for special occasions, but be sure to take them home with you when you leave.

If Mom is the sort of lady who has always loved wearing jewelry, and just isn't "dressed" without her earrings, by all means, bring a large assortment in for her to wear daily. I know my mom won't leave the house without her earrings, and if she ever goes to a nursing home, her jewelry will go with her. Then I will put a sign on the wall saying "please put earrings on daily!" so no one will be in any doubt about what she wants. Many aides are really very good about being sure their ladies are outfitted properly, as long as they know this is what the resident and the family want. If they forget - remember to "squeak!"

12. Safety and Restraints

Safety in the nursing home environment is one of those subjects that is of primary importance. Any building or environment - they just can't be safe enough. And when you are dealing with the elderly, it seems to be of even more importance.

I have tried to list a few things that can help any facility to be a safer environment.

Very few facilities have carpeting throughout. Some may have carpeting in a few rooms, but for the most part, floors are vinyl or tile. Carpeting is softer, absorbs sound better, and provides more traction under foot, but it also is harder to keep clean, and absorbs odors over a period of time. It is true that the newer carpets are vastly improved over the older ones, but they still cannot be kept as clean. So, good, old, slick flooring is pretty much the norm in most nursing homes, and after they have had their required waxing, they can be pretty slippery, to say the least.

Things to notice when visiting the facility in this area: when the floors are being washed, are there hazard or caution signs at both ends of the wet area? Are there hand railings along both sides of every hallway? (These aren't just for the residents - I have had occasion to grab for them, let me tell you!) If there are area or throw rugs in resident's rooms, do they have a latex or rubber backing to prevent slipping? If you are allowed to, and chose to bring in throw rugs or an area rug from home, be sure they have a non-skid backing of some kind. Falls are probably the primary injuries sustained in nursing homes. As we get older, our balance just isn't what it used to be, and if the flooring is slick, it can be an open invitation to a fall. If Mom actually does come to stay in a nursing home, be sure to remind her to use the hand rails whenever possible. Side rails on beds are another issue, with ardent advocates on both sides of the fence, so to speak. Some nurses and administrators don't want to ever see a side rail, while others think every bed should have them. Personally, I feel this depends on each resident individually. Often, even one rail up at night can really be a great assist for turning in bed, or even getting up. Today, side rails are considered a "restraint", and require a doctor's order to have them up at night, or any other time. Many residents feel safer with side rails up, and request this. (They often are afraid of falling out of bed.) If Mom wants both side rails, or even one up just at night, be sure to tell the doctor so he can write a specific order upon admission. It can work both ways, though. While for some residents side rails are a safety measure, for others, who may be confused, they can be a real safety hazard. I have seen numerous broken hips over the years, obtained by a confused resident crawling up over the side rails and out of bed during the night. It's farther to the floor if you go over the rails! So this is an issue that may need to be discussed with the resident, the doctor, and the nursing staff. The aides who are working nights can be of the greatest help in deciding which way to go with side rails. They are the ones who see Mom during the night the most frequently, and can probably give the best input as to which is the safest. Remember that every situation is different. But if Mom is one of those who definitely wants one rail up at night (usually the one against the wall) to help her turn over or get out of bed, stick up for her, and insist. Again, the old "squeaking hinge" theory. Check out the bathrooms when you visit the facility, the ones where the bathing is done. Are there hand rails around the walls? Are the tubs easily accessible to people either ambulating or in wheelchairs? Are there "lips" on the edges of the showers, or can a wheelchair just roll on in there? Are there grab rails next to the toilets? (I can't imagine any facility today NOT having grab rails!)

Watch the aides and nurses transferring residents who need assistance - are they grabbing the residents under the armpits, or are they using "gait belts"? Gait belts are wide, nylon webbed safety belts that the resident wears for transfers. The person doing the assisting holds onto the belt rather than the resident's arms, and is a much safer method of transferring anyone. These are indicated for everyone, but especially for residents with osteoporosis or arthritis. If you see nurses or aides transferring residents without them, ask them why the belts aren't being used. If they say it is not facility policy, I would question as to why it isn't, and seriously consider placing Mom somewhere else where they ARE used.

Check the beds in resident's rooms. Unless they are beds brought from home, they are probably older hospital beds, and they all have small wheels with locks on them. See if the wheels are locked - they should be. If the bed rolls freely, ask the nurse why the wheels aren't locked. The only time the wheels should be free is if someone is actually moving the bed for some reason. Another one of those good fall prevention things!

Are there call lights in every room next to every bed? Every resident should have a call light in reach when in his/her room, and especially when in bed. The call lights can be clipped to the pillow or the bedding if necessary, and it is simply unacceptable for any resident to be in bed with no call light within reach. Just another one of those little things to sort of notice as you stroll down the hall on one of your inspection tours! And when Mom does take up residence in a facility, be sure the call light is one that she can operate easily. Some people have disabling conditions, such as rheumatoid arthritis, and special adaptations may be necessary. To be sure, explain the call light to her, and have her demonstrate that she understands what it is for and is able to easily to press the button.

I mentioned that side rails are considered a restraint - well, so are "posey vests", wrist restraints, and numerous other devices. Simply tying a "sash" around Mom while she is in a wheel chair, to prevent her falling out of it by leaning too far forward is considered a restraint, and cannot be used without a doctor's order. If you notice a lot of residents in the facility wearing these "sashes" around their waists, ask the nurse why they are being used. Personally, I think they are great. The elderly tend to doze off at any hour of the day, and they can topple right out of a chair - any chair, wheeled or not! To me, it is a sign that nurses and aides are paying attention to their residents, and doing the best they can to prevent accidents. I realize that there are those who would disagree with me on this, but again, I have seen too many accidents to feel otherwise.

Posey vests are really pretty neat little vests that some residents wear at night to prevent falling out of bed. They can turn over to either side, but the "tails" of the vest are tied to the bed frame, and the resident, while able to move pretty freely, cannot roll out of the bed. They are seldom used, but they are really great for the confused resident that tends to crawl out of bed during the night, and might easily fall. Another thing to be discussed with your doctor if confusion is a factor. If Mom is pretty confused, and you and the doctor agree that one of these vests might be an intelligent thing for her to wear at night, be aware that accidents can still happen. I have never seen a restraint yet, including Posey vests, that some residents can't get out of. There are some real "Houdinis" out there, genuine escape artists that can literally crawl their way out of anything. Just remember, again, that accidents can still happen no matter how hard you try to take all necessary precautions.

Are the halls free of clutter? Laundry carts, believe it or not, can be the cause of a fall. If they are left out, a resident walking down the hall may have to try to walk around the cart, and end up with nothing to hold onto but the cart itself, which has wheels, and away they go! They will be in the halls during rounds, but when rounds are over, the carts should be stowed away somewhere out of sight, and for sure out of the halls.

Wheelchairs are another thing that should never be left in a hallway, for the same reasons, but are a common sight in some facilities. (But if you do see a few sitting around, be sure to notice whether or not they are clean, while you have the chance!)

If you notice a lot of clutter in the hallways, and you are concerned, don't hesitate to ask someone why the halls aren't clear. They may not like the question, but it might make them think!

Be aware, though, that accidents will happen, no matter how hard the staff tries to prevent them. Most facilities try their best to prevent them, but sometimes their best is never enough. If you see something that you feel may be a hazard to either the residents or the staff, be sure to tell a nurse or the administrator. They will probably thank you for your suggestion.

13. Incontinence

One of the most dreaded aspects of getting old is incontinence. However, just because we don't like it, we can't always avoid it. As one ages, the elasticity of the bladder tissue decreases, and this is just a fact of life. It doesn't necessarily mean that we all become incontinent, but a large number of us will. It for sure means that we can't wait as long between potty stops, because the bladder simply will no longer hold as much.

This is a subject that I have very strong feeling about. Can't help it. So I will be very opinionated here, and since I am writing this, I can say whatever I want to! (This is great! I can finally speak my mind!)

Odds are, if Mom isn't incontinent when she enters the nursing home, she will become so in time. It may be that she would get to this stage even if she stayed at home, but it can also be directly related to the nursing home experience. Sorry, but I really feel that this is true. Why do I feel this way? Several reasons.

First of all, I think I have mentioned "time" before. Time is critical in the nursing home - there is simply never enough of it for the staff. Because the facilities are in business to make money, the staff to resident ratio is kept to the bare necessary minimum, usually whatever the state requires and no more. The smallest home I ever worked in had only thirty residents, and two or three aides on at a time, depending on the time of day. Usually there were three on in the morning, and two in the afternoon. There was also an LPN on duty during the day. Now if none of the residents required two people to assist them, that meant that each aide had ten residents to get up and dressed every morning, and then to the dining room. Most people don't like to get up too early, so that means that everyone is wanting to get up at essentially the same time. Now you know yourself, when you first awake in the morning, you immediately need to go to the bathroom, and depending on your age, (and what you had to drink the night before!) sometimes you can't get there fast enough. Well, imagine a hall full of residents all wanting to go to the bathroom at the same time, and no way for them all to get there when they want to. It is a physical impossibility. And sometimes, when you get that old, you just can't wait. So what happens? You wet the bed. You can't help it. And it really isn't anyone's fault, there just isn't enough help right at that time. Do that enough times, (wet the bed) and you become incontinent. I have seen it happen often enough to be pretty sure I am correct in this assumption.

Another culprit, I feel, is the standard medication, Lasix. If you have ever taken the medication yourself, then you know what I am talking about. I took it for years before I was smart enough to ask my doctor for an alternative medication. Let me explain for those of you who have no experience with it.

Lasix is a very strong diuretic, and works directly on the kidneys. Now for some people, there is no alternative, because nothing else will work as well. About twenty minutes to an hour after taking the medication, you have to go to the bathroom. And I mean you have to go NOW! It becomes a whole lot more than just an urgent feeling, it can actually be painful. I was in my thirties when I took it, and there were a few times I thought I might literally explode, because I couldn't get to a bathroom. (Once I was in an ambulance, transporting a patient who was having a heart attack. There are no potty stops in an ambulance for the nurse! I'm not sure who was in worse shape, to tell you the truth-me or the patient we were transporting!). Anyway, it isn't just one trip to the bathroom, either. Every twenty minutes for one to three hours, you have to go, and again, you have to go NOW! For someone who can get themselves to a bathroom, it is merely an inconvenience. But imagine if you are elderly and require help getting to the bathroom - you are in big trouble! Lasix is one of the most common medications taken by the elderly - sometimes up to half or more of the residents in a nursing home are on Lasix. And it is usually given at the same time for everyone, that time being at eight o'clock in the morning. That means that everyone who has taken Lasix will have to go to the bathroom at approximately the same time, and again, there just isn't the staff to get them all there when they need to go. And they will all have to go again in another twenty to thirty minutes. And maybe again after that. It just can't be done, and in all probability, someone is going to be incontinent.

Aides become very frustrated over the situation, because they don't understand what is happening. I personally think that a lesson in some medications should be given to every aide when they start work, but that is not the case at the moment. So they don't understand the mechanics of what is happening to all these residents. And because THEY don't have to go to the bathroom every twenty minutes or so, they don't understand why Greta and Hilda and Frank and George all seem to have to go to the bathroom so frequently. I have heard them tell residents "I just took you to the bathroom not twenty minutes ago! You CAN'T have to go again already!" They are not being cruel, they don't know that Greta and Hilda and Frank and George all took Lasix at the same time, about an hour ago.

So what can be done about this situation? Not much, I'm afraid, but I do have a couple of ideas.

First, talk to Mom's doctor, and request a different medication for fluid retention other than Lasix. There are some out there. It may be that Mom's condition is severe enough that Lasix is the only one that will work effectively, and if that is the case, there is not much to be done about it. But if another one will work, beg for a trial run. Also, Lasix depletes the potassium in the system, thus requiring a daily potassium supplement. It also means monthly or every few months a blood test to determine if the potassium level is where is should be. (More cost, and more pain for Mom). There are other diuretics that are potassium sparing, and thus the need for a potassium supplement is eliminated, as is the severe urgency problem in many cases. Study up on different medications, so you will be knowledgeable when you speak to the doctor. Ask your pharmacist for whatever information he can give you, or maybe he can assist you in where to look. Most pharmacists are more than happy to help with any questions you may have.

If the doctor simply won't change Mom's Lasix to another medication, you will have to deal with the problem as best you can. One way is to be sure there is adequate protection if Mom develops a "leakage" or incontinence problem. I worked in one facility where they used cloth "diapers" for the problem. These are totally unacceptable, in my opinion. They get wet, and there is no waterproof protection for their clothes. Residents end up sitting in wet clothing, which means more laundry and more inconvenience for the residents as well as the staff. It looks bad, it smells bad, and it is an indignity for the resident to endure. Some facilities provide Attends undergarments, but many do not. If they aren't provided, and you can afford them at all, they are well worth the money spent for this problem. (Attends are the equivalent of modern disposable baby diapers, and they are great!) There are other generic brands available, which are probably cheaper, but remember that often you get what you pay for. If you can't change the medication, maybe you can get the nurses to change the time it is given. (Nurse's are the ones who generally set the times for medications to be given. Occasionally the doctors will set specific times, and some meds MUST be given at certain times to be effective.) If everyone else is getting their Lasix at eight o'clock in the morning, ask if Mom can get hers at ten o'clock, or two o'clock instead. Maybe if she can be excluded from the majority in this way, the aides will have a better chance of getting her to the bathroom when she needs to go.

The other solution is to hire a private personal care attendant to come in for a few hours every day. Not only would the attendant be responsible for taking Mom to the bathroom as needed, but she would also be responsible for making sure Mom is dressed appropriately, has her make-up on, her jewelry on, her hair fixed, etc. She could also be responsible for the bath, which means probably more time could be taken as needed for a more pleasant bathing experience. I realize this is an added expense, but I have seen families do this, and it worked great. Sometimes family members simply took turns doing this themselves, to save money.

Remember, though, if Mom becomes incontinent (for whatever reason) sometimes it is just a fact of life, and there is nothing you can do about it. Don't be shouldering any added blame for yourself, because it might happen under the very best of circumstances.

Sometimes families think catheters are the solution to the problem. (I know most nurses and aides love that idea!) However, most doctors are very reluctant to place catheters because of the risk of bladder infections, which is the most common problem with them. And bladder infections can be very nasty indeed. I have seem some go undetected, and the resident can end up with a life threatening systemic infection. Mom may stay cleaner, but it just isn't a healthy alternative to the problem.

By the way, if it is only a minor "leakage" problem, incontinence pads may be the only thing you need. These are available at the drugstore. Or sometimes panty liners designed for heavy menstrual flow will work wonderfully. Check them out.

Just keep in mind that incontinence is really a pretty natural occurrence with the elderly. It is nothing to be ashamed of, but it can be dealt with.

14. Resuscitate/DNR/Living Will/Etc.

Here we go with a subject that many people don't like to discuss, and some refuse to discuss. But it is one of the most important topics I feel I need to cover, so I am going to spend a little time in this area.

Every facility has a form that needs to be completed upon admission, called a DNR form. (It may be called by other names, depending on the facility, but the topic is the same.) Usually it is a nurse on duty that does the admission, but it could be someone from a different department. They may broach the subject in different ways, but again the topic will be the same.

The question to be answered is, "If Mom's heart were to stop beating, and she also stopped breathing, do you want us to perform CPR and call the ambulance?" Sounds like a simple enough question, but it really isn't. Many people don't have any idea what the question actually means, so I will try to explain.

What we are talking about here is actually the absence of life. No heartbeat. No respiration. This is clinical death. Now, while it is true that often, for younger people who are found in the first few minutes of this condition, CPR can be successfully performed, the same is NOT true for the elderly. People watch programs like "ER", take CPR classes, and end up thinking that CPR is great, and most people can be saved. Let me repeat, this is NOT true.

Remember, we are talking about elderly people here. For many of them, especially those with osteoporosis, doing chest compressions while performing CPR will undoubtedly result in most of their ribs being broken. Bones become more fragile as we age, and they fracture much more easily. Chest compressions are done with force, and elderly bones just can't take that kind of pressure without breaking. Should a miracle occur and with CPR the individual is actually revived, the quality of life for the elderly person is often almost nothing. It is so rare that they are able to recover with no loss of function that I frankly don't even like to mention it as a possibility. I have seen a few "successful" codes, and let me tell you, they were very nearly comatose. I have NEVER seen an elderly person coded with full return of previous functions.

I think we have to remember that aging and death are natural functions of life. We can minimize our risk factors of an earlier death and debilitating quality of life, and we may be able to prolong death for a time, but we cannot ever eradicate it. We are all going to die sometime. I think the important thing is to make the latter years of our lives and those of our loved ones as comfortable as they can be. For the elderly person, CPR can, at best, prolong life for a short period of time, and at worst, remove any quality of life for that person, reducing him or her to little more than a vegetative state. I personally never want to exist this way, and I doubt that many of you do either.

So please, discuss this subject with your family members while they are still able to comprehend what you are talking about. I have never met an older person that wanted CPR performed, should the need arise, once they really understood all that it entails. Actually, I have met very few YOUNGER individuals that wanted the procedure. If you and/or your loved one do not want CPR performed, ever, be sure to talk to your doctor and sign a form stating your request. It isn't legal to just tell your relatives and your doctor - there must be a signed form on record somewhere, cosigned by your physician. When I was in nurse's training and this subject came up, I was most upset because I NEVER want it done to me, under any circumstances. I even questioned whether or not it would do any good to wear a medical alert bracelet with my wishes engraved on it, or as a last resort, could I have "NO CPR" tattooed across my chest. I was informed that the legal document is the only way my wishes would hold up, should the occasion occur. Remember that once you have "died", it is a little late for you to tell people what you want done! Do it now. I advise this for EVERYONE.

Some confusion exists between a Living Will, and a No CPR order. Many people think that if they have a living will, they have covered all the bases in this area - NOT TRUE!!! A Living Will only states what measures you want should the needs arise. For example, if you are no longer able to swallow, do you want a feeding tube placed? Do you want IV's for hydration, or for administration of pain medication only? Do you want continuous oxygen administration? These are all areas that you have choices in, but they are also conditions that can be planned ahead for. They generally cover conditions that occur rather gradually. CPR, however, is a split second decision. If, for example, an aide walks into Mom's room and finds her unresponsive on the floor, with no pulse and no respiration, the decision whether or not to perform CPR must have been made previously. If there is no "DNR" (Do Not Resuscitate) sheet in the chart, by LAW the aide must start CPR and do all she can to revive the resident. DNR does NOT include situations such as choking. I have run across more than one family member who firmly wanted CPR done because they thought that if a resident simply couldn't breathe, we would just let them lie there and die. Of course not! Their heart is still pumping, and we would do the Heimlich maneuver, as well as anything else that could be done, to revive them. CPR is only in question if there is NO pulse and NO respiration. Both conditions must be present before CPR would be initiated.

So please, please, please, talk to your loved one before the need arises. Talk to your doctor. If you decide that CPR is not for Mom (or for YOU, for that matter) fill out the necessary paperwork. And upon admission, bring a copy to the nursing home to put in the chart. I really think that this is one of the best things you can do for your loved one. There is such a thing as death with dignity, and we need to remember that.

15. Power of Attorney

Power of Attorney (POA) is another area that people seldom think about. And when they finally do, it can be pretty difficult to accomplish. At the present time, I am 50 years old, and I gave my best friend POA several years ago. I have had lawyers caution me, asking whether or not I really trust my friend. After all, she could sign documents and clean out my bank account or something. Or even worse, for me, load up my horses and sell them, and keep the fortune they might bring! (That's a joke in case you were wondering.) In my case, if I can't trust Myrna, I can't trust anybody, and she can just keep my POA.

In the nursing home situation, POA is pretty handy to have. If Mom gets really sick, and can't make her own decisions or carry on her own business in any way, if she has already given you POA there will be no disruption in her affairs, as you are already in position to make decisions without consulting her. As long as you both get along, and trust each other, I think it is one of the best things you can arrange before entering the nursing home. If a general POA is unacceptable to Mom, ask her to consider a POA for healthcare only. While you couldn't make financial transactions and decisions for Mom, you WOULD be able to make healthcare decisions for her with no difficulty. For instance, maybe when Mom entered the nursing home she had a living will in place that stated she would want a feeding tube placed if for some reason she was unable to swallow. But now, she is unable to communicate, and it is obvious that a feeding tube would only prolong an uncomfortable situation. She can no longer tell you that she doesn't want the tube, but you feel she really wouldn't want it in this case. With a POA, there is no problem, and you can make the decision.

There is another little known area that POA could possibly effect. Most people are not aware that their charts (hospital or nursing home) are legal documents. Every little thing done to the person involved is supposed to be charted somewhere, and for sure every medication and major procedure, as well as complete descriptions of any accidents. Every person has the right to read his/her own chart if they so desire. Now, normally, there is no reason to ask to see a chart, but every now and then, a question arises that reading the chart could possibly clear up. If you have Mom's POA, you have access to her chart without getting an attorney and a court order. I don't want to open a real "can of worms" here, but with a little imagination, you can probably come up with some scenarios where you just might want to read the chart. Here's a simple example: Mom had some blood work done, and you want to know how the tests came out. You ask the nurse and she tells you that everything was within the normal range, and not to worry. Fine. Everything is normal. But remember that for most lab values, there is a range, so there is "high normal" and there is "low normal". If Mom is borderline in some area, for example her potassium, and she is taking good old Lasix, her potassium level should be rechecked in a week or two. It is possible that the doctor as well as the nurse may not catch it, reading only the "normal" part. It never hurts to ask to read the lab reports, and if you have questions as to what they mean, ask the nurse. If Mom is getting physical therapy for a broken hip, perhaps, sometimes reading the therapists report can be more enlightening than talking to the therapist (if you can catch up with her!)

I definitely do not want to encourage family members to be reading their loved one's charts indiscriminately, or just for reading material. This is a waste of everyone's time, and just not necessary. But again, should the need ever arise.

16. Job Descriptions: Who Does What?

It might be slightly helpful to quickly explain just what it is that the different departments do in a nursing home. Housekeepers might get upset if you asked them to help transfer Mom to the commode, and aides might give you a blank look if you asked them what time Mom took her last Tylenol. So, before you make an embarrassing mistake, let me try to describe just what the various jobs are.

First of all, I really think that all personnel should wear large, easy to read name tags that show what department they are in. For instance, "Kathryn Miller, RN." Or "Sam Johnson. Housekeeping". I have seen more than one male aide wearing a stethoscope around his neck after checking on a resident, approached by a family member and asked, "Doctor...?" Name tags can make life SO much easier, for everyone!

Nurses are responsible for medication administration, treatments, communication between family members and doctors, patient plans of care, and general monitoring of the resident's condition. They are also in charge of supervising the nursing assistants (or aides). It is my understanding that all facilities must have a Registered Nurse at least on call, depending on the size and classification of the facility. Otherwise, LPN's (Licensed Practical Nurse) are used as much as possible. (They are cheaper! Got to remember the budget!) Don't ever think that Mom is possibly getting short changed in the nursing department if she is seen only by the LPN's. Some of the best nurses I have ever worked with are LPNs. When I was in the hospital myself, on one occasion it was the LPN who was really on top of things, and gave me the best nursing care. But in the nursing home, unless they are doing "primary care" the nurses, whether RNs or LPNs, are usually only doing medications and treatments.

It is nursing assistants, or aides, that provide most of the "hands on" care of the residents. They are the ones that really make a nursing home run properly. I have never felt that these people arc paid nearly enough for the work that they do. It is the aides who see the residents at all times. They are the ones that the resident's tell when they are in pain. Or, if the resident is unable to communicate, because the aide has been working with him/her regularly, they can tell when something is out of the ordinary. Good aides can pick up on a slight change in no time. They inform the nurse, and action is taken. It is the aides that give the residents their baths, brush their teeth, take them to the dining room, change their beds, take them to the bathroom, listen to their stories, fix their hair in the morning, and become like family to them.

Housekeepers keep the facility clean. It is also amazing what housekeepers observe. I have had more than one come to me with a concern about a resident, for good reason.

The Director of Nursing oversees all the nurses and aides. She makes out the schedules, hires and fires, and in general does a lot of paperwork that helps keep the facility "legal" with the state. She usually does very little hand's on care, so if you have a question about Mom, don't go to her if you can help it, unless it is a small facility.

The Administrator oversees the management of the entire facility. All the different departments report to him, and he takes it from there. He generally knows next to nothing about the condition of the residents, but if you have a problem that hasn't been resolved, or a billing problem, I would go directly to him.

Activities people are responsible for seeing that Mom makes it to church, if she wants to go, for getting her involved in exercise class, crafts, etc. She also makes notes in the chart commenting on what activities Mom participates in, and how she interacts with others.

I have skipped over dietary, purchasing, lawn care - maybe some others I have forgotten about. But the facility cannot operate for long if any department is missing. No one department is more important than another. (Sometimes they get a fat head and THINK they are more important, but it just ain't so!) Just as your hand won't work as efficiently if you are missing some fingers, so a nursing home won't function without all its staff. So, don't ever look down on anyone because they aren't a nurse, for example. And please don't ask the nurse or the aide to clean the toilet if it is dirty, either!

But if you want to know how Mom slept last night, ask the aide taking care of her. If you want to know what the doctor said about her latest "episode", ask the nurse. If you want to know why your bill is $500 more this month than last month, talk to billing personnel or the administrator. If you want to know how Mom interacts with other residents or how she spends her free time, ask the activities person. If you can't turn the faucet off in the bathroom, have someone page maintenance. You get the idea!

17. The Little Things?

I have discussed some of the "Big Things", like cleanliness and what to look for in that area, and now I want to address some of those "little things" (depends on who you are, and where you are, as to how "little" they are!)

By now, you have Mom in the nursing home of your choice, and you hope that all is well. It probably is just fine. But if you REALLY want to know how things are going, I will discuss some of those little things that are often overlooked in a facility, but to me are extremely important for the quality of everyday life in the home.

Baths. Facilities always have a bath schedule, and Mom will be on there somewhere. It might not hurt to check the schedule and see when her bath days are. If you can't find it, ask an aide or the nurse, and they can look it up for you and tell you what days she is scheduled for. In most facilities, baths are given twice a week. Bathing too frequently can be very detrimental to the elderly, as our skin tends to dry out considerably as we age. So don't be upset that Mom is bathing only twice a week - any more than that really isn't very good for her. But as always, there can be a problem.

If Mom is able to communicate, be sure to ask her if she had her bath. It might be a good idea to visit on bath days, when the experience would still be fresh in her mind. Of course, if you visit on her scheduled bath day, you ought to be able to tell just by looking at her if she had one or not. Why do I mention this? Because, going back to the big MONEY subject, sometimes the facility is short handed, and if there isn't the personnel there to do all the required tasks for the day, obviously something is going to get skipped. The nurses and aides will prioritize, in that instance, and the least important aspects of care will be the ones not done for the day. Bathing heads the list of these non-essential tasks, and Mom might only get one bath that week. Now, getting only one bath for one week surely won't mean the end of the world, and worse things can happen than that. The trouble is, if the family doesn't monitor the situation, it is possible that more than one bath might get skipped. I have seen this happen. I know of one instance where the resident did not receive a scheduled bath for three weeks. This is unacceptable! But unless someone is actually tracking the bath schedule, it can happen. Again, the old "squeaking hinge" principle comes into play. Staff listens to family. Always. They may not always like it, but they do listen. You can tell, if you visit, whether or not Mom had her bath. If you suspect that she didn't, find a nurse, (skip the aide in this case) and ask the reason why no bath was given. If you get the "run around", or she tells you there just wasn't enough staff that day, I would get upset, and question WHY there weren't enough aides on to give all the baths. That will put the nurse on the spot, when it really isn't her fault, but the Director of Nurses, or the Administrator. However, if the staff knows that YOU know, and you are upset, the chances of it happening again are greatly reduced.

The evening back rub with lotion is another little task that is more often than not neglected, again for the sake of time. There is just never enough of it for the aides, it seems. Upon admission, I would be sure to ask whoever is giving you a tour of the facility and answering questions for you whether or not the evening back rub is policy in that facility. If it isn't, it certainly should be, and you should request that one be given to Mom every night when she goes to bed. In all fairness, I have worked with some aides who are so very conscientious about this, it is a pleasure to walk into a room after they have settled someone down for the night. After a good back rub, the resident sleeps better, and the whole room smells somehow fresher after the use of lotion and sometimes powder. But often, this little task is overlooked in the rush. And if you are wondering whether or not the back rub is being given, and the aide or the nurse tells you it is, check and see if there is lotion at the bedside, maybe in the drawer. If there isn't any there, Mom isn't getting her nightly back rub, for sure. They are never given without lotion, so it is simple math - no lotion, no back rub. Ask the nurse. It isn't critical, but one of those nice things that, if possible, you should try to monitor for Mom.

The aides are required to pass fresh water to every room at least once a day, and usually twice. There should be a fresh pitcher of water, and definitely a clean glass or water bottle at the bedside at least once a day. Again, a little thing to sort of check on when you visit. If the glass or bottle is pretty "groaty" looking, you might question whether fresh water was passed that day. This is another thing that you can raise a little squawk about, but often it is easier to just go to the kitchen, or the dining room, or wherever in that facility, and get fresh water and a clean glass yourself. But if you suspect that the water isn't getting passed regularly, again, speak up! Tell the staff about it.

I mentioned wheelchairs earlier, and if Mom is using one, when you visit, check it over to be sure it is clean. If it is crusty, speak up!

If you brought jewelry in for Mom, and when you visit you notice that she is never wearing any, mention to the nurse that Mom really would prefer to be wearing the things you brought for her. You could tell the aide, (always a good idea!) but in this case, if you tell the nurse it should be noted and passed on to all the different shifts. Hopefully the next time you visit, Mom will be more cheerfully decked out!

If Mom had a favorite television program, or a certain schedule for, say, writing letters or taking a nap, be sure to let the nurses and aides know about it. It may not be possible to follow her routine from home at the facility, but if at all possible, the staff will try to the best of their ability.

Another thing - and to me this is extremely important. When you bring Mom in, be sure to let the staff know of any specific physical things, such as in what position she prefers to sleep. For example, my mother was in a car accident while visiting in England years ago, and while she didn't actually fracture her hip, she is unable to lay on her left side for longer than about twenty minutes. If your loved one has a favorite sleeping position, or is unable, like my mother, to sleep in a certain position, be sure the staff knows about it. Maybe she needs a pillow behind her back at all times while in a chair? Does she have one knee that gives her trouble if it isn't elevated while sitting, with a pillow under it? If Mom is able to communicate with the staff and let them know how she is feeling, this probably isn't quite as important as for those residents who cannot express themselves. If in doubt, again, let the staff know Mom's special needs in this area, and it never hurts to make a sign and put it on the wall in the room. A sheet of plain notebook paper, with the message written in big black letters will work just fine.

I realize that life is never going to be like it was at home for Mom, but honestly, the staff does really try to make it as pleasant as possible for the residents. Sometimes they get so busy with the big things, that the little things get lost in the shuffle. It is seldom intentional, but sometimes they just don't realize that some of the little things have been missed, because they aren't life threatening.

18. Mind Tapes

Here I go, off on another one of my tangents and pet subjects. In nurse's training, we studied geriatrics just as intensely as we did obstetrics. And one of the main things I was taught was reality reorientation for the confused and disoriented. We were taught that when we went to see Mrs. Smith to give her ten o'clock medications, for example, if we see that she is just staring out into space, we are supposed to have a conversation with her that goes something like this: "Good morning, Mrs. Smith. How are you doing this morning? (Mrs. Smith ignores us, and continues staring, unblinking.) Do you know what today is? (No response.) Today is Friday. It is the fifteenth of July. It is a beautiful day outside today, and maybe we can take you out for a spin in your wheelchair later this afternoon. Would you like that? Mr. Clinton is our president. You are in the Sunny Valley Retirement Home, and this is your room. Your family will be in to visit this evening." And Mrs. Smith just continues to ignore you.

Now, maybe my instructors were actually correct in teaching us to reorient these people on a daily basis, and I guess it doesn't hurt. But if they go to activities, they usually get a full dose of that sort of thing there, anyway, so why keep repeating it? The main thing is, who really cares?

Lest you think I am being really callused about this, let me explain why I feel the way I do. You see, I have my own memories that I have stored away, mostly the very best ones, and I call them my "mind tapes". I have stored them specifically for playback at later times. As we get older, we naturally start to accumulate life experiences, and thus memories. The more we get, the more we store. As we get older, I think a lot of us purposely "make tapes". We recognize an event as one that we want to keep with us as long as possible, so we start that little camera in our heads for specific shots we want to keep. I know I for sure do this, and if I do, I suspect a lot of other people do also. (I know I am weird, just ask my kids and they will verify that fact for you! But I don't think I am THAT weird!) I don't really consider myself to be that old, but I have days even now, when I can sit in my chair and just "leave" for a couple of hours at a time. I am playing my mind tapes. And it is a pastime that I am enjoying more and more as I age. I love to do it. And do you know what? I really get UPSET if someone interrupts a particularly good tape I am playing in my head. I am there because I ENJOY being there, and I prefer to be left alone.
So, I naturally reasoned, if I play my mind tapes for relaxation and enjoyment, how many others are doing the same thing? And how many of those elderly people sitting in their chairs, staring out into who knows what, are actually just replaying some of their favorite mind tapes, and having a wonderful time? And then some stupid nurse walks in and tries to bring them back to reality. Now I ask you, would you prefer to stay fishing on that mirror finished lake with your beau, in the summer of 1939 when you were young and beautiful, (or handsome, whatever the case may be) with the birds serenading you and the sun on your face, or do you want some idiot to come in and remind you where you are and who is president?

So why do we automatically presume that these old people who are just staring vacantly are miserable? Why do we feel so sorry for them, especially when we visit a nursing home? Just because they don't live the same type of lifestyle that we do, does that mean that they are unhappy? We aren't there yet, and we can't really understand. But I know that if I ever go to a nursing home, I will be playing a LOT of tapes. I am going to tell my children to pass the word on to the staff to just leave me alone, because I have a lot of tapes that need playing, some of them over and over again. Don't feel sorry for me and don't try to reorient me - I am happy where I am. And if I am old enough to be in a nursing home, I really don't care WHO is president! Just get me to the bathroom when I need to go, and to bed when I want to sleep. And of course, keep the food and coffee coming!

19. Family

I cannot overemphasize the importance of family in the overall nursing home experience. If you haven't guessed already, I think family is probably THE most important factor in the quality of nursing home life. The staff can only do so much, and they will do generally the very best that they can. But they are there to primarily take care of physical needs, and often emotional needs can go unnoticed. That is where family comes in.

The happiest residents I have ever seen in facilities, on the whole, were those whose families visited regularly, and by regularly, I mean usually daily. It doesn't have to be a spouse, or a daughter - it can be anyone. Cousins, grandchildren, friends, children - you name it. Remember that the nursing home is now THEIR home, and treat it as such. Did Mom have a lot of company while she was at home? Then keep it up! Let her friends know that they are welcome to visit any time.

Keep in touch any way you can. If you can't visit as often as you would like, if Mom is able to use the telephone, have one installed in her room and keep in touch by phone. Get her a cell phone if she is willing and able to use one. If it is long distance for you, send her just a short card every week. You would be appalled at how few letters are received in nursing homes, and there is no excuse for that.

Why not come in and have lunch or supper with Mom once a week? I know of one young man that came weekly to have lunch with his mom, and she really looked forward to it. Check at the nurse's desk or in the kitchen before hand and see what it will cost, then be sure to let them know when you will be coming so a place can be set for you. The cost is usually very nominal - usually only a dollar or two. Or, if you can't take the time for lunch, stop in for coffee. The kitchen will usually supply some cookies for you too, or toast.

Encourage the grandchildren to visit. This is harder to do, as they always seem to be so busy with their own lives, but the smile it puts on Grandma's face is priceless. If you have to, don't make it an option - tell Sally to visit her grandma or else! Another visitor that all resident's love to see is a baby. Any size, any shape, any color, any age, they love babies. I remember when I was in college, (way back when, in the dark ages!) I was walking downtown one day and happened to see some children playing in the park. All of a sudden it hit me - there were no children or babies on campus, where of course I spent most of my time. Now, I admit I have never been one of those people who make over babies, but I found that I actually was MISSING seeing children and babies. They are a part of the natural world, and unless families make an effort to visit, the elderly in nursing homes are deprived of that aspect of normal life. So, if there are children and/or babies in the family, please bring them in to visit. It can be more educational to the children than you would ever dream, and I know what it does for residents!

I have mentioned the "squeaking hinge" on more than one occasion, previously. Being a nurse and having been the recipient of that "squeak" more than I care to remember, I can tell you that I don't like it. There were times when I really hated to see a certain someone approach me, because I knew there was going to be another complaint lodged. "Why didn't Mom get her bath today?!" "Mom's teeth didn't get brushed last night and they are filthy." "I just checked, and Mom is wet again - why hasn't she been changed?" One gentleman came daily to visit, and at least once a week he came with a list of things for the nurse that he felt should be done for Gracie. None of us liked to see him head our way with a piece of paper in his hand. But you know, he always apologized for making trouble before he started on his list, and I knew that he was only trying to make the nursing home environment the best it could possibly be for his wife, who had Alzheimer's and was unable to communicate. I certainly understood what he was trying to do, and so did the rest of the staff. And you know what? Because he cared enough to take the time to come in and monitor his wife's surroundings, we took extra care to be sure things were done right for her. It may sound callus, but when the staff knows that the family really cares about their loved one, they seem to be a little more careful about what gets done, and when.

Another gentleman came in three times a day, at mealtimes, to feed his wife, who could no longer feed herself. We loved to see him come as he was always so cheerful and willing to help! He would help push wheelchairs to the dining room, and take residents back to their rooms after meals. When he was able to feed his wife, that left an aide or a nurse free to spend more time with another resident. And when his wife died, he continued to come in to visit other residents he had become acquainted with during his wife's stay there.

I know one really special young lady who had an aunt and an uncle in two different facilities. The uncle was in a regular nursing home/rehab center, and the aunt was in a personal care facility. She took it upon herself to take care of these old people, because they had no one else, and believe me, she did her job for them! She was in each facility at least three times a week, and she didn't just pop in, say "hello", and run out the door again. She spent time with each of them. She had coffee, she played cards, she took them for walks outside when the weather was nice. But brother, when something should have been done that wasn't, we heard about it! Loudly! I respected this young lady, big time. No one made her look out for her aunt and uncle, but she not only came to visit, she made it her business to know just what kind of care they were getting on a daily basis. And she wasn't afraid of anybody - if she didn't feel the care being given was up to par; she would chew out a doctor just as fast as an aide.

Those are the kinds of people I like to see in facilities. They are what keep the residents young at heart, and functioning. They are the lifeblood, so to speak, of the positive nursing home experience for these people, and I just wish more families were like that. I truly think that the quality of life in the nursing home is directly related to the amount of family involvement. Don't ever be hesitant to visit, to take notice of what is going on, to tell the staff what you think, to make suggestions, and to just be a positive part of the whole experience. It can be more rewarding than you ever dreamed.

20. Alzheimer's

Alzheimer's Disease is a horrible condition. It robs the individual, as well as the family, of a person's most prized possession - their mind. There is no cure, and no way of preventing it, that we know of today, and often, in the end, the nursing home is the only place for people with this condition to live. While physically they may be in great shape, mentally, they can't live at home anymore. They often require constant, monitored supervision, which just can't be done at home unless the family can afford to hire private help around the clock. Most of the larger nursing homes have special units for Alzheimer's residents, and I would like to discuss these units for a minute.

If you come to visit the prospective nursing home, and Mom has Alzheimer's Disease, you will get a tour of the Alzheimer's unit. This hallway is usually off by itself, with double doors separating these residents from the rest of the facility. Most families first impression is utter dismay when they enter the unit. The resident's are wandering aimlessly, often looking very unkempt. The beds may be torn apart in the rooms, there may be residents sleeping on the floor - it is often, in general, a very depressing area upon first glance. But please don't despair.

First of all, understand what is going on here. These people are in their own little worlds, and are often unreachable. Some can be violent at times, and must be handled carefully. Nurses and aides who work in these units have had special training. They know how far they can push a resident to participate in the routines of daily living, and how far they can't. On one of my first excursions to an Alzheimer's unit, I heard the most awful, loud screaming. I just knew someone was being tortured down the hall! And from the sound of things, I mean really tortured! I asked the nurse what on earth was going on, and her reply was, "Oh, it's Henry's bath day." She could tell I was skeptical, so she took me to the bathroom to let me see for myself. Sure enough, it was Henry's bath day, and he just wasn't having any of it. There he was, in a shower chair, screaming his head off while the aide was patiently lathering his back. This is a common occurrence, and happens frequently.

I later had occasion to work in Alzheimer units, and found them to be quite pleasant. Just remember that nurses and aides can't work miracles, and these residents will continue to live in their own world. I remember one gentleman that used to go down the hall and strip every bed he came to. It was terribly frustrating for the aides, but there just wasn't any way to stop him from doing it. Another man needed to wear oxygen at all times, but of course he wouldn't even consider it, and as a result was constantly exhausted. He would lie down on the floor whenever and wherever he chose, and took a nap. Rather than try to move him, we had to let him stay where he was. We would bring him a pillow, and sometimes we were able to at least slide him to the side of the hall, but it did look rather pathetic to visitors.

Remember that these people are not in pain, and they are not being abused in any way. They are just difficult to deal with, and the staff does the very best that they have been trained to do. They are never medicated unnecessarily, and their aimless wandering and vacant stares are not related to drugs. (Unless they are violent, in which case some medications may be used to prevent injury to the staff as well as other residents.)

21. Nurse Consultants

Nurse Consulting, in the nursing home environment, is a relatively new field. I have heard of it in some of the eastern states, but have no knowledge of where these nurses can actually be found. I thought of starting a business in my home state, but met with a lot of resistance from both state officials, and local home health agencies, as well as nursing homes and personal care facilities. Why? To explain this, let me explain what a Nurse Consultant actually does in the nursing home setting.

A Nurse Consultant is a Registered Nurse, or an LPN under the direct supervision of an RN, who is hired privately by either the resident or the family of the resident. The nurse goes in to visit the resident either weekly, biweekly, monthly, quarterly, or on whatever schedule the employer has set up. She does an independent assessment to ascertain the true physical condition of her client. She may check the medications being given, and assess their effectiveness. If authorized, she will go through the chart and determine if the plan of care is appropriate for the client. She may be a liaison between the family/client and the doctor. If given the authority, she will go over the monthly statement, and determine if services and supplies being billed for are actually being supplied. The Nurse Consultant is responsible only to her employer, and is actually employed as a patient advocate in every respect.

State authorities and facilities HATE these nurses, because they are the ones who can REALLY monitor patient care. For all the little things that can get lost in the shuffle of daily life in the nursing home, the Nurse Consultant will ferret out the discrepancies. I am not necessarily implying that the nursing care given in the nursing home is not up to par, but it is never the less true that in some cases it definitely is not. Sometimes the only way to find out is to hire an independent observer with a medical background to come in and actually check everything out. It is truly amazing what can be uncovered! Nurse Consultants, I think, are a must for the family that lives in another town or state from their loved one. If the family really wants to be sure that the best possible care is being given, they need somebody outside to come in and assess the environment. If everything is fine, she will inform her client. If it isn't, she will make a direct, concise report to the family, and the family can then ask for suggestions on what course of action to take, or proceed on their own.

Again, sometimes it's the little things that get missed in the nursing home. Maybe Mom has a history of congestive heart failure, and fluid may tend to accumulate in her lungs. It isn't that the nursing staff is necessarily being lax in their monitoring of their residents, but again, the old time factor comes into play. Often, they aren't listening to resident's lungs unless someone notices a problem - perhaps a chronic cough, or difficulty breathing. A Nurse Consultant, if she was going in weekly, would routinely listen to lung sounds and would be able to detect fluid retention in that area before the resident became symptomatic. She would then report to the family, and also contact the doctor directly, get the resident started on the proper medication, and possibly avert a bout of pneumonia and/or a hospital stay.

Maybe the family gets the monthly bill, and notices that Mom seems to be using a lot of disposable gloves. Or maybe the family DOESN'T notice that Mom is using that many gloves, but the Nurse Consultant catches the item on the bill, and realizes that eight boxes of gloves in two weeks just doesn't add up. It is a fact that in many facilities, supplies are often billed to residents other than the ones who actually using them. I have seen it happen, and it is done intentionally because "Mrs. So and So can afford it better than Alice. Just put it on her bill - she won't know the difference." And they arc right - Mrs. So and So DOESN'T know the difference. A Nurse Consultant WOULD, if she makes regular visits.

Now, obviously, the facilities aren't going to like this nurse coming in to check on Mom. She might find too much. She might question too much. The state doesn't like them because the nurse might, again, dig up some "dirty laundry", shall we say. Nurses don't like them, whether they be home health nurses or facility employees, because they see the Nurse Consultant as infringing on their "territory", so to speak.

But the beauty of the whole concept is, if you are interested in patient advocacy, no one can top a GOOD Nurse Consultant. They are answerable only to their employer, usually the family of the resident, and as such have no fear. They are free to do their jobs, and they do it well. Their schedules are their own, so they are able to make surprise visits any time they want. And since they are nurses themselves, they really know what they are looking for. They take pride in their work, and do it to the best of their ability.

So, how do you find one of these paragons of the nursing profession? Good question. You will have to look, but it can be done.

First of all, check the yellow pages of the local phone book. You might get lucky and find someone or an agency listed there. If not, try calling the state department of health - by some miracle they might know of someone who is doing this type of work. Talk to the local home health agencies. Again, someone may know someone who knows someone who does this kind of thing. Ask the office nurse at your doctor's office. Nurses know other nurses, and even if they don't know someone right off hand that does this type of thing, they may know someone who might be interested in doing it. You might check with the state board of nursing in that state - all licensed nurses are registered with that agency, and they may be able to help you. These nurses are out there, all you have to do is find them.

If Mom is in the facility for a period of time before you decide you want to hire a consultant, you can always ask one of the nurses employed at the facility. Get to know the staff, the aides as well as the nurses. Usually there will be one or two nurses that stand out in your mind that do exceptional work, you know, those individuals that are willing to go the extra mile for their patients, and genuinely have the resident's best interests at heart. These individuals, while not able to do the consulting themselves, may know other good nurses that would be willing to work in that capacity for you. Good nurses love their residents, and they will do whatever they can to help you provide the best possible care for Mom.

If you choose to hire a Nurse Consultant, I think that in the end you will be more than happy with your decision, especially if you happen to live a long way from the facility. She can save you a lot of questioning and soul searching, and possibly some money. Even if she only came in once a month, you will rest easier at night, knowing you arc doing everything you possibly can to provide the best environment and care for your loved one.

22. Abuse

I really debated whether or not I wanted to address this subject or not. We all hear about the occasional abuse episode, and we all know it happens at times. There are many different forms of abuse in nursing homes and personal care facilities, just as their are in marriages or other family environments. We know what the ideal is, and we know it is seldom reality. Let me say, to begin with, that although I HAVE seen physical and emotional abuse in the nursing home setting, I have NOT seen very much of it. Actually, considering how long I worked in facilities, I saw very little, overt or otherwise. And abuse is something that we as nurses are trained to constantly be on the look out for.

There are the accidents that possibly could be categorized under abuse, because they resulted from either carelessness or the staff just being in too big of a hurry. These usually manifest in the form of large bruises and skin tears, acquired while the resident is being transferred. But lest you immediately think Mom is being abused because she got a large skin tear on her forearm, please remember that the elderly have extremely fragile skin, and sometimes it seems that all you have to do to is look at them, and they bruise or tear. Some residents are just perpetually in a bruised condition, and no matter how careful you try to be, it happens. However, if you notice excessive skin tears that require steri-strips, or what you feel are excessive bruises, talk to the nurse and voice your concern. Again, staff listens to family!

A more subtle form of abuse may be just leaving a resident in a wheelchair too long at a time. Remember the old "Squeaking Hinge?" Well, residents use that principle also. The more vocal ones, who complain the most about wanting to lay down for their nap, are often the ones who get to bed the quickest, while the elderly lady who is unable to speak may have to sit there the longest because she is quiet. She doesn't com-plain. But she may be in the most discomfort. To me, that is a mild form of abuse.

Another "pet peeve" of mine, that to me is abuse, is the use of soup spoons while feeding a resident. I for one never use a soup spoon - they make me gag. Yet because of the shortage of staff in nursing homes, when residents have to be fed, aides will often use soup spoons, and heap them with food, in an effort to get the meal over with more quickly. I tried to gauge the response of the residents when they were being fed, and if it appeared that someone was not comfortable being fed with a soup spoon, I would ask the aide to use a teaspoon. If this affects you and your loved one adversely in some way, make your wishes known to the staff - NO soup spoons at meal time.

Sitting for too long in wet clothing, or wet "diapers" is another one. This can be a difficult area to monitor, because let's face it, an aide might have taken Mom to the bathroom ten minutes ago, and she didn't go, but she was dry. In that ten minute space of time, she has now wet herself, but you come in to visit and you have no idea how long she has been sitting there, wet. And yes, there are some lazy aides out there who will tell you they took her to the bathroom, or they just checked her and she was dry, but the reality is, they never did either one. So what do you do?

The best solution I found to this problem is to have the aide initial, date, and time the "diaper". They should all be carrying pens with them for charting anyway, so all they have to do is write on the edge of the plastic when the resident was last changed or checked. This practice, I found, tended to keep most of the aides honest, and some even took pride in being able to justify themselves and their work.

Not turning residents that cannot turn themselves at night is another form of abuse. Again, this goes back to lazy staff. Residents are to be turned every two hours if they are in bed, to prevent pressure sores. For the resident who is unable to turn, and it is not done for them, this can be a painful experience. One facility that I worked in put a paper clock on the wall, with moveable hands on the face. As each aide did her rounds every two hours, she moved the hands of the clock to show what time she was turned. On another sheet of paper, also taped on the wall, the aide put her initials, the time, and the position she left the resident in. If you suspect a problem like this, you might suggest the clock idea to the nurses. Maybe it will help.

Of course, to me, not getting my bath is a severe form of abuse!! And I feel it is also abuse for the residents who cannot bathe themselves,. I discussed this earlier, however, but I know that skipping baths happens. Again, seldom intentionally, but because of lack of time and manpower, it DOES happen.

Hitting and slapping happens. We all know that it does. But again, very seldom. An aide might get away with it for a short period of time, but there is almost always someone, whether another aide or a resident, who will suspect or actually see it happen, and reports it. Usually this kind of thing goes on at night, and if the staff member is changed to a day position, it usually stops because it can't be hidden. These people seldom stay long in one place. That doesn't make it any better, but there is no fool proof way to guarantee that this form of abuse will never happen. The staff does the best that they can to prevent it, and again, it truly is rare in my experience.

One form of abuse that I have noticed happens among the nurses. This is generally brought about by the Director of Nurses, when she is wanting her nurses (usually LPN's) to learn a new skill. They need to practice, of course, so who do they get? The residents that cannot speak for themselves. I remember one incidence where a resident had gone to the hospital for x-rays, and while she was at the hospital, the doctor called the nursing home and ordered an IV started. I immediately called the hospital and asked them to start the IV over there. I had drawn blood from this lady numerous times in the past, and while she wasn't hard to draw blood from, her one good vein would "blow" every time afterward. I knew that starting and maintaining an IV on her would be more than difficult. I am usually pretty proficient at starting IV's and could have done it if I had to, but I was soon leaving for the day. I may be proficient at starting IV's, but some people just need that special hospital IV team to start them. Anyway, to get on with my story - the Director of Nurses just happened to be at the hospital when I called to ask the team to start the IV over there. She told them not to start it, because the LPN's needed the practice. So she brought her back to the facility to start the IV there. When I was ready to leave for the day, I stopped in the resident's room to see how things were going. The resident was lying on the bed, tears running down both cheeks, both arms black and blue from the elbows down, nurses still trying unsuccessfully to start the IV. When I returned two days later, I asked the Director of Nurses how many times they had stuck the resident in order to start the IV, and she replied, "numerous". To me, this is abuse, big time. And it was my boss doing it. What is the point of this gruesome story? You might want to make it a point, upon admission, that if any IV's are ever to be started, or any procedures done in the future that require nursing skills, you DO NOT want any nurse "learning" on Mom! Make the point loud and clear. I realize that nurses have to learn some of these things somehow, and in some cases, only practice on a real live person will do. But in those cases, they can ask someone who is alert, oriented and able to speak for themselves if they can practice on them. It should NEVER be done on someone who cannot speak for themselves.

Do you know what I feel is the saddest form of abuse that takes place in nursing homes today? It is the lack of family involvement. To me, the resident that sits in her room day after day, never getting visits from home or from friends, neglected by family, is the most abused resident of all. You can take a lot from people if you know you have family support - you know this yourself. So again I say to you, please, please, please get involved in your loved one's new life at the facility. In the end, it really doesn't matter so much to anyone what is going on around them, if they are not cut off from all that they have always held dear!

Have I scared you now? I hope not. Again, I repeat, bad things do happen in nursing homes that sometimes we are powerless to prevent. But nurses and aides for the most part love their residents, often like their own families, and would never do anything in any way to hurt them. Abuse happens. But not often. And generally, everything that can be done to prevent it, IS done.

If you ever feel that there is some sort of abuse going on, you have reported it to the nurses, and then to the administrator, and you still feel that something is "just not right", call the State Ombudsman. His number should be posted in plain view in a prominent area of the facility. If it isn't, ask the office or the nurse for it. It is your right to call this person any time you feel there is a need, so don't be hesitant about it.

23. Angels

Now I come to the fun part of this whole thing. I have mentioned a lot of "bad stuff" that you need to be watching out for, but now I would like to, hopefully, renew your faith in mankind, and fill you in on some of the really "good stuff" that I have seen happen in various facilities.

I think I mentioned somewhere that most of the facility staff ends up loving the majority of the residents, and come to think of them as their extended family, and this is very true. But there are some outstanding examples of this.

There was one aide I worked with in two different facilities, at two different times. She was no kid, and was in her late fifties, but worked just as hard as any of the younger aides on staff. I think she suffered from arthritis, because she walked very stiffly, but she never complained. And if there were shifts that someone had called out for and we were short staffed, she was always there to fill in, even if she hadn't had a day off in more than two weeks. She couldn't say "no". But complaints always came back to me that Gertrude was slow in getting her work done. This was a constant complaint. But do you know why she was slow? All you had to do was quietly follow her around, which I did one day, to find out just what was going on. She was slow because she took all the extra time desired by each of her assigned residents. She took the time to fix their hair, rather than just quickly combing it. She took the time to put lipstick on her ladies before they left the room. She took the time to sort through their jewelry and find just the right accessories for them to wear before they went in public. She never rushed her people when she took them to the bathroom - she sat and visited with them if they wanted her to.

I remember when one of her favorite residents was dying. It was peaceful, but there was no one to sit with her the last few days. Her family lived out of state and were on their way, but wouldn't arrive for another two days. Gertrude came in every day after work and sat with this lady. Just sat with her. She didn't get paid to do this, she did it because she loved that old woman, just like family. Towards the end, she even came in during the night. I have no idea when she got any rest, but it didn't seem to matter. She was there.

Another aide that I worked with in that small nursing home was also older. Sometimes Vicki got a little flustered, and could at times be a little "short" with the residents, but she did her job well, and all the physical tasks were always done properly. I remember one resident in particular who was in his early seventies, and was profoundly retarded from birth. He had no family, and was a ward of the state. Without getting too graphic here, let me just say that Alfred was not the most lovable person by any stretch of the imagination. He was always dirty, because we couldn't keep his hands away from certain areas of his body. He couldn't talk, or feed himself, or communicate in any way. Alfred was an easy person to sort of forget until the last minute, and as you can imagine, he was not a favorite with the aides, because that man was WORK!!

One day, around nine o'clock in the morning, two representatives from the state showed up totally unexpectedly to check on their ward, Alfred. No one knew they were coming, and as I escorted them down the hall, I really was a little worried about how Alfred was going to look, especially that early in the morning. I was so proud of Vicki that morning, as we walked into Alfred's room. I don't think I had ever seen him looking better. He had been washed up, shaved, his eyes were clear and sparkling, his fingernails were clean (that in itself, for Alfred, was a major accomplishment!) and neatly trimmed. He had a clean, white tee shirt on, his hair was combed, and Alfred looked GOOD! Vicki was nowhere around at the time, and I didn't know who had taken such good care of him until later. Believe me, I checked, because I wanted to hug whoever had done such a great job that day. Needless to say, the state people were more than satisfied that Alfred was being well taken care of, and gave the facility a glowing recommendation. Vicki was good. And she loved her people.

I have found that in every facility there are those residents who are really lovable, and those that are not so lovable. There are those that can talk and act just like your grandma and grandpa, and those that don't communicate at all. Some seem to be always soiling themselves, no matter how hard you try to keep them neat and tidy, and others never seem to have a hair out of place no matter what happens. It is just the normal "range" of people, found I think, in any environment. And it is also true, just as in any environment, that people are attracted to different individuals, for whatever reasons. There are always those few really special residents that everyone just automatically loves, just as there are those few residents that seem to be totally unlovable. But for those that seem to be so unlovable, there seems to always be an aide who takes that resident under his/her wing, and loves them to death. Maybe it is because no one else does, I don't know. But I have a story I want to tell you about these unlovable residents.

In one facility I worked in, E-Wing was the location of the most heavy care residents. Most of these people required two aides to get them up and going for the day, and there were also some of the more belligerent residents on that wing. You know, those people who just can't get along with ANYBODY, in or out of the nursing home. Ida lived there, who more than once threw her morning glass of juice on me for who knows what reason. Jackie lived there who was another lady who liked to put fruit where fruit should never be put, and was NEVER clean. And there were several others that the aides just didn't like taking care of. These residents were always presentable in the dining room, or the lounge, but never more than that because since they seldom allowed more care to be taken with them, and the aides had long since stopped trying. Imagine my surprise when I started seeing these residents in the dining room, absolutely shining. Their faces were actually radiant on certain days. Jackie and Ida had their hair fixed, their makeup and jewelry on. Talk about rings on their fingers and bells on their toes! I was impressed. I didn't know what was going on, but after a couple of weeks I began to wonder. It only happened on certain days. So finally, I asked the nurse on that wing who was taking care of these people who were now looking so good. I wanted to compliment that aide, because whoever was doing such a fantastic job with such difficult residents needed to be commended! You cannot begin to imagine how proud I was when that nurse told me the aide responsible for those people was my son, Sean. Because of nepotism, we never worked on the same wings, so I wasn't aware of what kind of job he was doing.

When I questioned him later about his job performance, he told me that someone had to love those people, and he found them to be really lovable. It was no trouble for him to take the extra time with them. When I think of those residents today, it brings tears to my eyes, because SOMEONE thought those people were lovable. It just happened that that someone turned out to be my son. Who, I might proudly add, has since gone on to become an RN. But the point of the story is, no matter how repulsive you think a resident is, there is SOMEONE in that facility that loves them, and will go the extra mile for them.

I know of a nurse who routinely purchased personal supplies for residents out of her own pocket. She couldn't afford it, but she had the biggest heart! She never asked the facility to reimburse her for these expenditures, she just quietly purchased them. She also was available to take residents to the store, on her off hours, if they had no way to get there, and needed help in the store itself. This nurse really didn't have the time for this kind of thing, as she was married with two children, both of whom had special needs and required extra time.

I remember another lady who was very old, and dying. Again, slowly and peacefully, but the process just seemed to be dragging on. Knowing the woman was a strong Christian, the nurse asked one of the visitors that she knew played the piano if she would play some hymns so this woman could hear the music. The visitor was glad to oblige, and sat down to play hymn after hymn, all the old favorites. The dying woman had been unresponsive for about two days, but a smile came over her face as she heard the music playing in the hallway. That same nurse came in and sat with the woman, and read scripture to her in her off time. Again, no monetary compensation, just a good deed. There were two daughters of this same woman, both of whom lived out of town. One lived about forty-five miles away, and the other one lived out of state. Both were at the bedside as often as they could toward the end, but the drive back and forth from the closest sister's house was starting to wear on them both, as they weren't young themselves anymore. This same nurse went out of her way to talk with administration about letting the sisters stay upstairs in an empty room, to save them that long drive. The administrator went along with the idea, and they were able to stay in the same facility, free of charge until their mother died. Maybe a little thing, but to those sisters, an immeasurable blessing.

There was a resident, an elderly man who needed to be transported to a hospital by ambulance for surgery. The ambulance ride was about a two hour drive, and the gentleman was very arthritic, making every movement very painful for him. The nurse on duty that was arranging the transport, suddenly thought of the pain that ambulance ride would in all probability cause him, and called the doctor to request a shot for pain right before transfer, which the doctor did. However, the order was for a high dose of Demerol. Before the ambulance arrived, there was shift change, and the nurse leaving reminded the nurse coming on to give the injection about fifteen minutes before the gentleman left. The nurse coming on refused to give the injection, feeling it was too strong a dose, and might possibly cause the man some respiratory distress. (Translation, he was afraid the injection might kill him, which was nonsense!) Anyway, the nurse wouldn't give the shot. So the nurse that was leaving stayed an extra hour, off the clock, to give the injection. She didn't want her patient to go through that ride in pain. She didn't get paid. She just did it.

I have seen staff bring in books from home, plants, food, anything you can think of, actually. If they think they can help a resident in some way, there is always someone who will do it with no thought of reward.

I know another nurse that took it upon herself to distribute fresh coffee to residents in their rooms as they watched their favorite daytime programs. She just went around to the rooms, took orders for coffee and cookies, and brought it around. She didn't have to do that, it wasn't in her job description, but it was something that made life a little more pleasant in the facility.

The sad part is, staff comes and goes, but the residents stay. It seems like often, just when you really establish a fantastic relationship with someone, the staff member moves away or finds a better job. But you would be amazed at how many of these people go around the facility to say special good-byes to their friends, the residents. And when they can, they come back to visit, just like family.

In the end, that is what the facility ends up to be - family. It is a big home where family members all dwell together. Nurses and aides and housekeepers and maintenance people and cooks - they all end up spending time with their new friends and family. The younger members, when they start families and have children, are some of the first ones in the building showing off their babies. They bring their children in with them when they get out of school, to visit with the residents while they finish their shifts. And life goes on.

I know of another nurse who found "things" going on within a facility that she knew were wrong. Certain practices that she knew were being done were harmful to the residents, so she went through the chain of command in an effort to set things right. It's called being a patient advocate, something that we as nurses are all trained to be. I guess some just take it more to heart than others. Anyway, when she approached her supervisor with what was going on in several areas, she knew when the supervisor did not support her that her job might be in jeopardy, which turned out to be the case. The more the nurse refused to turn her back on the situation, and fight for the resident's care, the more she was discriminated against. In the end, the state was called in, but the nurse lost her job.

And then there are the REAL angels. Remember the lady I mentioned earlier with the two daughters? This woman had had a couple of strokes, months apart, about year before she passed away. She had mentioned seeing "men" in the room that no one else could see, and they were angels. One day, after the second stroke, one of the daughters came to visit her. She was talking with her mom, and asked her if she had seen the "men" again, to which her mom replied "Oh, yes. They're sitting right over there in the chairs!" The daughter turned to look, and of course no one was there - that SHE could see. But she told me that she sensed a holy presence, and had the immediate feeling that she was intruding on something. So she left. You will never convince her that there were no angels in that room! Her mom saw them. More than once.

My son also told me about a gentleman who was dying, and had not spoken in a day or so. He was extremely lethargic, and basically unresponsive. One evening when Sean went into the room, the gentleman spoke to him, saying, "Oh! Do you see them? The angels are here. They have come for me!" Sean looked, and again, there was no one else in the room. The gentleman died a short time later, peacefully. There are angels in nursing homes.

I could tell you lots and lots of stories about staff and residents, and the little miracles that take place daily in facilities, but you would get tired of reading it. Maybe that should be a topic for another time? As far as I am concerned though, there are some staff members who are nothing less than angels in human disguise. They go quietly about their business of providing the best care they possibly can for the residents, never expecting any more reward than maybe a smile from a grateful recipient. These are the people that really make life in a facility worth living. They are the ones, besides family, who put that smile on a resident's face in the morning upon arising, and in the evening when they are tucked in for the night. These are the people that let the world know there is hope for us as humans, after all.

A note from the author

I hope I have provided you with an overview of some of the things you might want to look for if you are considering choosing a nursing home for your loved one. I realize there are numerous other subjects that I could have discussed, but many of them would center around specific diagnoses of residents, and the individualized care that would accompany those situations. This was intended to be a simple guideline for choosing a facility, and then some of the things that can be done to make the nursing home experience all that it can positively be.

Remember, as I have said repeatedly, the nursing home environment is not necessarily bad - it is just different. There are little things that can be done to make the experience more positive - they aren't necessarily expensive, and they aren't difficult. But it's the "little things" that either make life more enjoyable or make it a massive headache for all concerned. And it's the families of the residents that really control the entire situation to a very large degree.

So, if Mom must go to a facility, she must go. But hopefully I have given you enough help and hope that the experience will be less fearful and more positive. Good luck!

art typing. Delete this text prior to use.

www.ingramcontent.com/pod-product-compliance
Lightning Source LLC
Chambersburg PA
CBHW051814170526
45167CB00005B/2006